Find a Way or Make a Way

Find a Way or Make a Way

Checklists of Helpful Accommodations
for Students with Attention Deficit
Hyperactivity Disorder, Executive Dysfunction,
Mood Disorders, Tourette's Syndrome,
Obsessive-Compulsive Disorder, and Other
Neurological Challenges

Leslie E. Packer, Ph.D

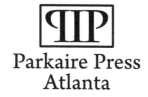

Parkaire Press
Atlanta

Published by:
Parkaire Press, Inc.
4939 Lower Roswell Rd.
Suite C-201
Marietta, GA 30068
www.parkairepress.com
info@parkairepress.com

Library of Congress Control Number: 2009901731

ISBN-13: 978-0-9818643-2-7

9 8 7 6 5 4 3 2

Printed in the United States of America

Cover photo by Dmitriy Shironosov. The child in the photo is a model.
Use of the photo is not intended to suggest that she has any of the disorders discussed in this guide.

Dedication

When educators approach accommodations not as a burden but as a creative challenge to find a way or make a way to deliver the curriculum,

When they have empathy and convey high hopes for the student,

When they model perseverance until the right accommodation is found and implemented in the right way and at the right time,

Our children flourish and begin to believe in themselves.

This guide is gratefully dedicated to three very special educators who each found a way or made a way to reach and teach my children:

Kathy Stock, Ann Katsaros, and Maria Abele

Leslie E. Packer, Ph.D.
February 2009

Table of Contents

Overview

Students with neurological or psychiatric disorders often experience significant academic, social, and behavioral impairment in school. To complicate matters, many children do not face just one challenge, but may have numerous diagnoses or features of a number of disorders. Trying to determine what accommodations or services any one student needs is often a daunting task.

Unfortunately, there is very little controlled research to guide us as to what accommodations work for particular problems as they relate to most neurological or psychiatric disorders. The National Center on Educational Outcomes maintains a searchable database on accommodations,[1] but searches for keywords such as Tourette, Attention Deficit, Bipolar, or other related diagnoses return no or very few results. Searching by type of accommodation (e.g., "testing") returns more results, but the testing accommodations may not be relevant or appropriate for students with the types of problems our children and students have. One of the best sources of information on what works, then, is often word of mouth from parents and teachers.

Although individualized accommodations are often necessary, creating a student-friendly environment by incorporating more visual and cognitive cues as well as consistent routines generally provides great benefit to a number of students and may reduce the need for individualized accommodations. In addition to specific problem- or diagnosis-related checklists, then, there is also a checklist for educators of helpful ideas that may reduce academic and behavioral problems in the classroom.

Almost 30 years ago, I saw a poster with a picture of a skier in a seemingly impossible situation poised at the edge of a glacial crevasse. The caption was "Find a way or make a way." I made that caption my personal motto, and invite readers to make it their motto, too, when it comes to helping students with disabilities learn and perform. Find a way or make a way -- around, over, under, or through their challenges.

[1.] http://www2.cehd.umn.edu/NCEO/accommodations/

How to Use This Guide

The first part of this guide provides a brief listing of the types of issues students with particular disorders may have in school. It also provides some screening tools or surveys to help parents and educators determine whether the student has handwriting, homework, or sleep issues that will need to be addressed. The three survey forms can be reproduced by teachers who wish to send them home to all parents towards the beginning of the school year. By screening for sleep problems, organizational deficits, and homework issues, teachers may intervene early with necessary accommodations and interventions, thereby preventing a lot of trouble. Parents can also use the forms to provide information to their child's teacher(s). Parents can simply complete the relevant survey and send it in with a note requesting a meeting to discuss the concerns and possible solutions.

The second part of this guide provides checklists of accommodations that might be helpful and necessary. The first three checklists address problem areas common to a lot of disorders, i.e., handwriting problems, homework issues, and the need for testing accommodations. Some accommodations in those checklists have qualifiers such as "If tics…. " or "If the student has handwriting rituals" etc.

The second part of Part 2 consists of checklists organized by specific disorders. Some parents and educators may not be familiar with the term Executive Dysfunction. Executive Dysfunction (EDF) is impairment in "getting your act together" (Denckla 2007). Students with EDF have trouble organizing, planning, following multi-step sequences, shifting flexibly, managing time, and using feedback, among other deficits. If you have ever thought of a child or student as "clueless" (Pruitt, 1995) or "terminally disorganized" (Packer 1995), the Executive Dysfunction checklist may be very helpful.

The disorder-specific checklists generally do not repeat the ideas for handwriting, testing, and homework that are covered in their own checklists, although there may be additional ideas specific to the disorder for those problems. In general, the diagnosis checklists focus on specific interference from the cardinal features of the disorder and what school personnel might do to accommodate the interference.

Most parents and educators will need to consult several checklists for any one student because most students do not have just one disorder or problem. If, for example, a student has Tourette's Syndrome and there are concerns about handwriting, homework issues, and testing that underestimates knowledge, the student's team may need to refer to all of the individual checklists for problems and then also consult the checklist for Tourette's Syndrome for more accommodation ideas for tics. If the student also has obsessive-compulsive symptoms with the Tourette's Syndrome, then even though they may not have full-blown Obsessive-Compulsive Disorder, the team may need to consult the OCD checklist.

The checklist for Attention Deficit Hyperactivity Disorder may seem surprisingly short given the complexity and seriousness of ADHD's impact on school functioning. Most of what are typically considered accommodations for ADHD are actually accommodations for Executive Dysfunction, however, and that is where those accommodations will be found – in the Executive Dysfunction checklist.

The second part of this guide also includes accommodations for other issues such as medication side effects and sleep problems, and a checklist for educators and administrators about classroom layout and other factors that if implemented classroom-wide or building wide, will result in a classroom and school that works for more students.

The third part of this guide provides a planner to help parents organize their concerns about their child's school functioning. School personnel may wish to encourage parents to use the form if the student is having a lot of problems and a meeting is planned.

Part 1
Identifying Areas of Concern

Identifying Areas of Concern

All of the disorders included in this guide have been linked to dysfunction in a group of brain structures (the Basal Ganglia) that regulate learning, behavior, and motor control. Students with one Basal Ganglia-related disorder often have features of one or more other Basal Ganglia-related disorders. Knowing what accommodations to try depends, in part, on our explanation for a particular problem. As one example, Attention Deficit Hyperactivity Disorder, Tourette's Syndrome, and Obsessive-Compulsive Disorder are all associated with handwriting problems, but the handwriting issues are different for each and require different accommodations.

Table 1 lists some of the major types of impairment associated with each of the disorders in this guide. The table does not represent a complete list of all known impairments for each diagnosis, but will give teachers and parents a starting point for considering whether the student may need accommodations for a particular issue.

Table 1: Impairment Due to Disorders

Tourette's Syndrome

• Handwriting impairment	• Distraction due to efforts to suppress tics
• Difficulty copying from board	• Peer rejection
• Fine motor control deficits	• Slowed reading due to tic interference
• Build up of frustration, fatigue, irritability over the course of the day	• Homework problems due to handwriting or build-up of frustration, tics, and fatigue
• Distraction due to tics	

Obsessive-Compulsive Disorder

• Handwriting rituals	• Memory deficits
• Difficulty copying from board	• Difficulty making transitions
• Impaired concentration due to intrusive thoughts and/or mental rituals	• Attendance or lateness problems due to rituals or anxiety
• Written expression deficits (when Executive Dysfunction is present)	• Task or setting avoidance due to obsessions or compulsions
• Number obsessions or compulsions, if present, may interfere with math	• Homework issues due to compulsiveness and impaired concentration
• Peer rejection or social problems	

Non-OCD Anxiety Disorders

• Impaired concentration	• Avoidance of tasks or settings
• Impaired performance on tests due to high anxiety	• Attendance issues or lateness
• Difficulty making transitions	• Peer issues (neglect, rejection, bullying)
• Cannot complete tasks in "normal" time due to interference	• Avoidance of social situations

Attention Deficit Hyperactivity Disorder (also see Executive Dysfunction)

- Handwriting impaired
- Coordination impaired
- Difficulty copying from board
- Difficulty sustaining focus
- Learning disabilities in written expression, math calculations, reading, and spelling
- Accident-prone or injury-prone
- Behavior and peer problems
- Oppositional behavior
- Working memory impaired
- Makes careless errors
- Speech and language problems (Inattentive subtype)

Executive Dysfunction (usually does not occur in isolation)

- Impaired planning
- Difficulty with big projects
- Written expression deficits
- Poor time management
- Fails to complete tasks
- Difficulty with multi-step sequences
- Failure to self-monitor
- Impaired organization
- Does not have or appreciate long term goals
- Difficulty making transitions
- Failure to use feedback
- Impaired Working memory
- Impaired social skills

Mood Disorders

- Impaired memory (especially in depression)
- Difficulty concentrating
- Difficulty accurately interpreting facial expressions (Bipolar)
- Difficulty with big projects
- Heightened impulsivity (mania, hypomania)
- Math difficulties (Bipolar)
- Moves slowly (psychomotor retardation of depression)
- Impaired planning

Asperger's Disorder

- Motor clumsiness
- Impaired handwriting
- Difficulty with inferences
- Difficulty with abstractions
- Difficulty making transitions
- Impaired social skills
- Difficulty empathizing with others
- Stiff or inappropriate facial expressions and gestures
- Hyperfocus on restricted interests

Homework Observations and Concerns Survey – Parent Reporting Form

Student's name: _____

Completed by: _____ Date: _____

ITEM	NEVER	RARELY	SOME	OFTEN	ALWAYS
My child records all of his or her homework assignments independently in school.					
My child brings the homework planner or recorded assignments home.					
My child brings home the books or materials needed to complete the day's homework assignments.					
My child misplaces or loses school work or homework.					
My child knows and understands the assignment(s).					
My child knows when the assignments are due.					
My child starts homework without reminding or nagging.					
My child leaves homework assignments until the last minute or is late in doing them.					
My child completes the homework without someone sitting with him or her.					
My child can shift or switch easily between homework assignments.					
My child packs up his/her school bag independently and correctly.					
The level of the homework is too difficult for my child to complete independently.					
The amount of homework is too great for my child to complete due to other factors (disabilities, after-school sports, medications, sleep problems, etc.)					
How often do you fight with your child about homework?					

How much time are you spending each day with your child on homework? _____

How much time does your child usually spend doing homework each day? _____

Add an additional page if you have additional homework concerns.

Organizational Skills Survey – Parent Reporting Form

Student's name: _____

Completed by: _____ Date: _____

ITEM	NEVER	RARELY	SOME	OFTEN	ALWAYS
My child keeps his/her bedroom well-organized and neat.					
My child misplaces or loses personal possessions, including favorite belongings.					
My child is always late for everything, even with reminders.					
My child knows what he is supposed to do each day.					
My child has a good sense of what is important and what is not.					
My child meets responsibilities in the home without reminders.					
My child makes social plans with peers in advance.					
My child starts non-school activities or projects but does not finish them.					
My child has trouble getting started on activities without assistance (do not include homework in this category).					
My child is a follower more than a leader.					
My child can follow three-step directions without forgetting one of them (e.g., "Turn off the lights in your room, come downstairs, and feed the dog.").					
My child remembers to give me notices from school.					

Other concerns about organizational issues:

Sleep Survey

Student's name: _____

Completed by: _____ Date: _____

ITEM	RESPONSE
How many hours of sleep does your child usually get each night of the school week?	
What time does your child usually go to bed on school nights?	
What time does your child usually fall asleep on school nights?	
What time does your child usually wake up for school?	
Once your child falls asleep for the night, does he sleep through the night or is sleep interrupted?	
Does your child wake up easily in the morning?	
Do you struggle to get your child up on school mornings?	
Does your child stay up late at night to do homework?	
Does your child sleep in the afternoon after school? If yes, for how long do they sleep?	
Does your child maintain the same sleep pattern on weekends or when school is closed for vacation? If "no," how is their sleep cycle different? _____	
Does your child set an alarm clock and wake themselves up in the morning?	
Other sleep related problems:	

Part 2

Checklists of Accommodation Ideas

Handwriting Accommodations Checklist

	General Accommodations
	Reduce amount to be handwritten at any one time. Indicate maximum _____
	Provide a movement break or opportunity to step out of classroom after every _____ minutes of handwriting.
	Reduce copying from the board. Indicate maximum _____
	Provide a movement break or opportunity to step out of classroom after every _____ minutes of copying.
	Provide copies of board work.
	Extend time for _____ handwritten work _____ note-taking _____ copying from the board. Indicate how much extra time as percentage of normally allotted time: _____
	Provide copies of class notes and lecture notes. Indicate whether _____ full or _____ partial notes will be provided.
	Do not grade for neatness.
	Provide a scribe for the student. Indicate whether the scribe will be used for _____ all or _____ some of the writing activities.
	Allow student to dictate notes into a recorder.
	Allow student to use computer/keyboard as an alternative to handwriting.
	Allow student to decide whether to use printing or cursive or keyboarding.
	Provide access to a computer in all academic courses.
	Provide student with _____word processor or _____laptop computer for _____ classes and for _____ home use.
	Provide special paper to accommodate handwriting (e.g., wide-lined, graph paper, vertical lines, greater workspace for math calculations, etc.). Indicate: _____
	Provide agenda or planner that leaves adequate space for student's handwriting.
	Provide pencil grips or wider writing utensils.

	Provide and teach use of voice dictation software (e.g., for students with severe motor tics but no vocal tics or for students with handwriting rituals).
	Allow separate time for editing handwritten work.
	Provide testing accommodations for handwriting (see Testing Accommodations Checklist).

When Handwriting Interferes with Calculations	
	Use _____ graph paper, _____ lined paper turned sideways, or _____ ruler guides to help student line up the numbers. Make sure that the graph paper fits the size of the student's normal writing.
	Modify worksheets to allow more space for work.
	Reduce number of problems to be done at one time.
	Fold, block, or mask worksheet so that student sees only one problem at a time.
	Allow separate time for editing.
	Modifiy materials for homework. Indicate: _____

Use the Space Below to Indicate Other Handwriting Accommodations	

Notes:

1. Has the student been evaluated by an occupational therapist? If requesting an assessment, ask that the evaluation include having the student produce a writing sample comparable to what is expected in daily class work and under similarly timed conditions to see if the student's handwriting is adequate to keep up with production demands. A dictated sentence test is not adequate.
2. Some students may need assistive technology. Request an assistive technology evaluation to find out what type of hardware and software the student needs in school and for use at home during homework time. If the student needs assistive technology, also arrange for training in the use of the hardware and any software. If the student will be using keyboarding, does the student need training in keyboarding skills? If so, be sure to include that in any plan.

Homework Accommodations Checklist

	General Accommodations
	Extend time for completing assignments. Indicate: 1.5x_____ 2x _____ other: _____
	Do not penalize for lateness.
	Reduce number of math problems to be done in one evening. Indicate: _____
	Provide special writing paper for _____ written and _____ math work.
	Allow use of calculator.
	Provide worked examples at top of math homework sheets.
	Reduce or modify reading assignments. Indicate:_____
	Reduce the number of times spelling words are to be copied. Indicate:_____
	Provide extra set of books to be left at home.
	Provide books on tape for homework.
	Allow student to use word processor or computer. School to provide _____ word processor or _____ computer for home use.
	Provide agenda or planner that leaves adequate space for student's handwriting.
	Alternative system for recording homework required: _____ Student will type assignments into computer or word processor. _____ Student will orally record assignments into recorder, computer, or voicemail. _____ Other system required. Indicate _____
	Have teacher or aide ensure that all assignments are recorded completely and accurately.
	Have teacher or aide ensure homework sheets are marked with "H" or some designated symbol at top of page and that the due date is written at the top.
	Have teacher provide back-up access to assignments via: _____ web _____ email _____ other: _____

	Have teacher or aide ensure that all necessary materials are packed for homework.
	Limit time spent doing homework to _____ maximum daily, for all subjects combined, including long-term projects and studying for tests.
	Have teachers coordinate so that student does not have more than one test to study for per night.
	Have teacher chunk big projects into smaller units with intermediate deadlines.
	Have teacher monitor progress towards intermediate deadlines on big projects.
	Have teacher provide weekly feedback to parent via _____ phone _____ email as to any outstanding assignments.
	Have teacher meet weekly with student to review any missing assignments.
	Provide parent with copy of explanation and instructions for big projects.
	Modify or reduce homework during periods of medication adjustment.
	Modify or reduce homework if sleep problems interfere with homework completion.
	Allow student to _____ fax or _____ email homework back to school.
	Verbally cue student to turn homework in.
Use the Space Below to Indicate Other Homework Accommodations	

Notes:

1. Use the homework survey in this guide to identify concerns.
2. Homework needs to be at the independent level for the student.
3. Some educators may be concerned about not penalizing for lateness, but grades are intended to reflect what the student has learned and accomplished. Penalizing a letter grade for lateness creates a misleading impression about what the student has actually learned and produced. Also, students who are going through symptom exacerbation cycles or medication changes may not be able to complete homework even with what may seem like reasonably extended deadlines. If penalized for lateness, the stress may further exacerbate their symptoms, produce demoralization, and lead to them shutting down and not trying at all.
4. Notifying parents of missing homework assignments by use of a communications notebook or note is not included because some students fail to bring the notebook or notes home. Using phone or email is more likely to result in the parent actually getting the message.

Testing Accommodations Checklist

Setting Accommodations

	Test in a separate location. Indicate location: _____ Indicate student : teacher ratio: _____ Proctor must be known to student _____ yes _____ no
	Test in separate location for: _____ quizzes _____ tests _____ district- or state-mandated assessments
	Have student: _____ start quiz or test in classroom and then continue in separate location _____ take entire quiz or test in separate location
	Allow the student to decline the accommodation at their discretion and take the test in the classroom? _____ yes _____ no
	Provide study carrel in classroom for quizzes.
	Provide larger table so student can spread out papers.

Time Accommodations

	Extend time. Indicate: 1.5x_____ 2x _____ other: _____ Applies to _____ quizzes _____ class tests _____ state-mandated tests
	Permit movement breaks during testing. Provide _____ minute break after every _____ of testing.
	Provide proctor for movement breaks during tests.
	Break up tests. Do not test for longer than _____ at one time, including movement breaks. Do not test for more than _____ in one day, total, including movement breaks.
	Allow separate time for editing (writing mechanics).

Scheduling

	Use flexible scheduling. Indicate time of day for important tests: _____
	Do not schedule more than _____ test(s) per day.

	Test Presentation
	Provide oral testing as alternative for following subjects: _____
	Clarify test directions.
	Read questions to the student.
	Check for comprehension of directions.
	Color highlight operational symbols in math tests.
	Color highlight test directions.
	Provide multiple-choice format as alternative to items requiring writing.
	Hand student only one part of the test at a time.
	Responses
	Provide a scribe.
	Provide extra scratch paper or work paper.
	Allow the student to dictate answers into recorder.
	Allow the student to _____ circle answers in test booklet and/or _____ record answers directly in test booklet.
	Allow the use of calculator.
	Have teacher or aide ensure that answers are copied over correctly to answer form.
	Provide word bank.
	Do not use computer recording (Scantron) forms.
	Have teacher mark correct answers (i.e., do not put an "X" through incorrect answers).
	Allow student to use word processor for responses longer than: _____
	Provide special paper to accommodate handwriting (e.g., wide-lined, graph paper, vertical lines, greater workspace for math calculations, etc.). Indicate: _____

Miscellaneous	
	Allow student to use white noise filters, baseball cap, or headphones to block out distracting noises.
	Do not penalize for spelling unless it is a spelling test.
	Allow student to retake test, without grade penalty, to demonstrate mastery. Indicate number of times student may retake quizzes or tests: _____
Use the Space Below to Indicate Other Testing Accommodations	

Notes:

1. If a student has Tourette's Syndrome and their tics worsen under testing conditions, the student's team can determine necessary setting accommodations by comparing the student's performance when they take quizzes under timed conditions in the classroom to: (a) taking quizzes with extended time in the classroom, (b) taking quizzes in a separate location with no time extension, and (c) taking quizzes in a separate location with extended time. Some students with Tourette's may not benefit grade-wise from testing in a separate location, but may need testing in a separate location if they have vocal tics that distract peers during testing. Under such conditions, help the student understand that they are not being punished and that the accommodation is designed to protect their peer relationships. If the student resists the accommodation (and some do) or if the parents resist the accommodation (and some do), the team, parents and student need to meet together to discuss how to handle the issue in a way that is both fair and sensitive to both the needs of the student and the needs of the other students.

2. Breaking state-mandated tests up over days or limiting the number of state-mandated tests given in any one day may require special application or state approval. In New York, for example, if students need a limitation on the number of Regents to be taken in one day, the district must apply to the state for that waiver/accommodation three months in advance.

3. The National Center on Educational Outcomes has a database of research studies on testing accommodations at http://www2.cehd.umn.edu/NCEO/accommodations/

Executive Dysfunction Accommodations Checklist

Difficulty Setting or Appreciating Long Goals

	Provide student with outline for lecture material.
	Provide syllabus.
	Review previous material and skills sufficiently and relate to goals before introducing new material.
	Relate new concepts and skills to concrete meaningful examples.

Difficulty Planning Projects

	Provide project planning template.
	Show student an example of completed project when first introducing project or assignment.
	Have teacher chunk big projects into smaller units.

Difficulty Organizing Materials and Papers

	Use color to organize texts, folders, and workbooks (i.e., consistent color for topic or subject).
	Use pocket folders or _____ other type of folders for filing papers.
	Assist student with organizing and cleaning out binders or folders on a _____ daily or _____ weekly basis.
	Assist student with organizing and cleaning out desk on a _____ daily or _____ weekly basis.
	Assist student with organizing and cleaning out locker on a _____ daily or _____ weekly basis.
	Allow student to keep an extra stash of supplies in classroom(s).
	Provide extra set of books to be left at home.
	Provide backup system available for obtaining homework assignments. Indicate: _____ web site _____ email _____ homework helpline _____ other: _____
	Allow student to fax or email homework back to school.
	Have the teacher or aide ensure that homework is recorded completely and accurately.
	Have the teacher or aide ensure that materials for homework are packed up.

	Have the teacher or aide ensure that intermediate deadlines are entered in agenda.
	Have the teacher conference weekly with student concerning missing or incomplete assignments.
	Have the teacher _____ call or _____ email parent each week concerning missing or incomplete assignments for _____ classwork and/or _____ homework. _____ Copies of missing assignments to be sent to parent.

Difficulty Following Multi-Step Sequences

	Place a math sequence of operations strip on student's desk .
	Provide cognitive cues for sequence of long division (e.g., "Does McDonald's Sell Burgers?" for Divide, Multiply, Subtract, Bring down).
	Provide mnemonic for editing written expression (e.g., "CLIPS" for Capitalize, Leave space, Ideas complete, Punctuation, Spelling). Place reminder on students desk.
	Allow separate time for checking or editing work (math, written expression).
	Check for comprehension of directions.
	Conference with student after first step to check for understanding.
	Provide first step and then pause before providing second step during orally presented directions.

Difficulty Making Transitions [1]

	Note changes in routine on the board and call attention to them.
	Cue changes in routine verbally.
	Stand close to student during unexpected transitions.
	Pre-warn student of routine fire drills.
	Allow more time for transitions.

Difficulty with Time Management/Pacing

	Externalize time: _____ Use countdown clock on their desk _____ Program devices for reminders _____ Provide verbal reminders or cues
	Establish multiple (intermediate) deadlines for big projects.

[1]Many students cannot make transitions simply because they have never been directly taught how to make a transition. Before providing accommodations, ensure that the student has received direct instruction in how to make transitions.

	Ensure intermediate deadlines are entered in agenda.
	Have teacher monitor progress towards intermediate deadlines on big projects.
	Allow more time for classwork.

Difficulty Getting Started on Tasks	
	Clarify directions.
	Check for comprehension.
	Stand near student at outset of activity.
	Conference with student after first step to ensure that they are doing it correctly.

Difficulty Sustaining Focus	
	Break tasks down into smaller units.
	Provide opportunities for movement.
	Use preferential seating: _____ facing area of instruction _____ close to teacher.
	Seat student next to good role model in terms of work pace and sustained focus.
	Tackle most difficult concepts early in the day.
	Provide _____ self-monitoring form and _____ reward system.
	Use teacher-directed instruction for new material.
	Use computer-assisted instruction to enhance focus.
	Use more self-paced activities.
	Use more multi-sensory activities.

Difficulty Prioritizing	
	Cue with "This is important."
	Student to be provided with _____ partial or _____ full notes for lectures.
	Provide _____ daily and _____ weekly prioritized to-do lists.
	Provide syllabus.

	Have the teacher or aide indicate homework priorities in agenda.
Difficulty with Written Expression	
	Place editing strips on student's desk with symbols that remind them what to check (e.g., spelling, punctuation, capitalization).
	Provide mnemonic for editing and place visual reminder on desk (e.g., "CLIPS").
	Allow extra time for written expression. Indicate: 1.5x: _____ 2x: _____ other: _____
	Allow separate time for editing.
	Provide _____ visual organizer (e.g., mindmap) and/or _____ visual organizing software to help student develop ideas for _____ classwork and/or _____ homework.
	Use one template or mindmap system in all courses requiring written expression.
Difficulty Inhibiting	
	Reduce environmental triggers to impulsive or disinhibited behavior. Indicate: _____
	Establish predictable routines.
	Allow more self-paced activities.
	Have student cross out wrong answers instead of circling correct answer.
	Allow larger buffer zone around student.
Use the Space Below to Indicate Other Executive Dysfunction Accommodations	

Notes:

1. Also see Homework Accommodations Checklist.
2. Executive Dysfunction (EDF) usually does not occur by itself. It is often comorbid with Attention Deficit Hyperactivity Disorder, Obsessive-Compulsive Disorder, Autism Spectrum Disorders, and traumatic brain injury, to name but some conditions.

Tourette's Syndrome Accommodations Checklist

	General Accommodations
	Do not comment on tics publicly.
	Allow the student to _____ leave the classroom to "get the tics" out in private and/or _____ to take a break in the classroom if the tics are becoming overwhelming. Identify where the student will be permitted to go: _____ (to be determined in collaboration with student)
	Allow movement breaks or opportunities to leave the room to discharge tics in private after every _____ minutes of work and/or _____ at the student's discretion.
	Allow student to _____ read for pleasure and/or _____ engage in an academically-related and engrossing task as a tic break (to be determined in collaboration with student).
	Allow student to _____ to reduce their tics if the tics are causing pain (to be determined in collaboration with student).
	Allow student to work in whatever position they feel most comfortable.
	Use preferential seating. Teachers to consult with student about where they feel most comfortable.
	Assist student with refocusing.
	Provide any information missed or copies of notes if tics distract student during the lesson or student is out of the room for a tic break.
	Break class assignments into smaller units.
	Allow student to avoid non-essential settings that are particularly stressful or where tics may distract or annoy peers (such as the library for students with loud vocal tics). This needs to be at the student discretion. Indicate those settings here: _____
	Provide staff development program for school personnel: _____ teachers _____ administrators _____ aides _____ related services providers Also include: _____ cafeteria personnel _____ bus personnel _____ other: _____
	Provide peer education program for: _____ classmates _____ all students in grade _____ entire building _____ other: _____ To be provided by: _____ (name) To be provided by: _____ (date)

© 2009, Leslie E. Packer, PhD.

	Schedule heavy academic courses for _____ morning _____ afternoon, if possible.
	Reduce or modify homework. Indicate: _____

Specific Accommodations During Class Work	
	Extend time on reading assignments.
	Use books on tape.
	Have someone read to the student.
	Allow oral recording or keyboarding as a substitute for handwriting.
	Consult with student privately about whether to call on them for reading aloud or speaking in front of class.
	Allow larger buffer zone or space around student.
	Provide second desk or alternative work area in classroom that student can use when tics are bad.
	Excuse student from specific tasks or activities if tics pose safety issue. Indicate: _____
	Provide added adult supervision due to safety issues. Indicate: _____
Use the Space Below to Indicate Other Tourette's Syndrome Accommodations	

Note:

Because tics wax and wane and new tics may emerge over the course of the school year, the accommodation plan may need to be revised.

Obsessive-Compulsive Disorder Accommodations Checklist

General Accommodations

	Do not comment on compulsions publicly.
	Allow student to leave the classroom or to take a break if they are "stuck" obsessing or engaging in compulsive behavior. Identify where the student will be permitted to go: _____ (consult with student as to "safe place")
	Use preferential seating. Consult with student about where they feel most comfortable.
	Assist student with refocusing.
	Provide any information missed due to impaired concentration.
	Give student prior notice and reminders of upcoming transitions.
	Provide added support for transitions (e.g., close proximity).
	Remove or avoid specific triggers, if possible. Indicate: _____
	Allow student to avoid settings: _____
	Allow a larger buffer zone around student.
	Provide staff development program for school personnel: _____ teachers _____ administrators _____ aides _____ related services providers Also include: _____ cafeteria personnel _____ bus personnel _____ other: _____
	Do not penalize for arriving late to school (see Note 1).
	Establish a check-in ritual when student arrives at school. Describe: _____
	Allow student to call home. Indicate frequency or contingency: _____
	Provide peer education program for: _____ classmates _____ all students in grade _____ entire building _____ other: _____ To be provided by: _____ (name) To be provided by: _____ (date)

	Reduce or modify homework. Indicate: _____
Specific Accommodations	
	Reduce amount to be read at any one time. Limit to: _____
	Extend time for reading. Indicate: 1.5x: _____ 2x: _____ other: _____
	Have someone read to student.
	Provide books on tape.
	Limit amount to be handwritten at any one time. Indicate: _____
	Set aside separate time for editing written work.
	Provide hard copies of lecture notes. Indicate: full notes: _____ partial notes: _____ .
	Fold, block, or mask worksheet so student sees only one problem at a time.
	Modify math work to avoid specific number(s): Indicate numbers to avoid: _____
	Allow use of calculator.
	Extend time on classwork. (see Note 2)
	Modify or reduce classwork to only give student as much as they can reasonably accomplish for the available time.
	Give student only one part of assignment at a time.
	Check for comprehension of orally provided directions.
	Mark correct answers (do not put "X" through incorrect answers).
	Assist student with any locker issues.
	Assist student with any _____ bookbag _____ desk _____ locker issues.
	Provide added adult supervision due to safety issues. Indicate: _____

Use the Space Below to Indicate Other Obsessive-Compulsive Disorder Accommodations		

Notes:

1. If the student is arriving late to school or avoiding school due to OCD, the student may require a behavior plan and/or treatment plan.
2. Extending time may enable the student to engage in compulsive behavior even longer. Consider how much extra time to allow.
3. Many students with OCD will need accommodations for Executive Dysfunction as well as for handwriting, testing, and homework. The student's team may wish to consult those checklists.

Non-OCD Anxiety Disorders Accommodations Checklist

General Accommodations

	Extend time on classwork.
	Allow student to leave the classroom or to take a break if student is highly anxious. Identify where the student will be permitted to go: _____ (consult with student as to "safe place" or "safe person") Specify if any limits on how often student may leave: _____
	Use preferential seating. Consult with student about where they feel most comfortable.
	Assist student discreetly with refocusing.
	Provide any information or notes missed due to impaired concentration.
	Give student prior notice and reminders of upcoming transitions.
	Provide added support for transitions (e.g., close proximity).
	Provide staff development program for school personnel: _____ teachers _____ administrators _____ aides _____ related services providers Also include: _____ cafeteria personnel _____ bus personnel _____ other: _____
	Do not penalize student for arriving late to school (see Note 1).
	Provide peer education program for: _____ classmates _____ all students in grade _____ entire building _____ other: _____ To be provided by: _____ (name) To be provided by: _____ (date)
	Modify or reduce classwork to only give student as much as they can reasonably accomplish for the available time.
	Give student only one part of assignment at a time.
	Check for comprehension of orally provided directions.
	Reduce or modify homework. Indicate: _____

Specific Accommodations

	Allow student to bring transitional object from home to school (for separation anxiety).

© 2009, Leslie E. Packer, PhD. 29

	Allow student to bring transitional object from school to home (for separation anxiety).
	Allow student to call home. Indicate frequency or contingency: _____
	Establish a check-in ritual when student arrives at school. Describe: _____
	Cue student to use relaxation techniques (see Note 2). Specify type of technique: _____
	Cue student to use cognitive interventions to reduce anxiety (see Note 2). Specify type of intervention: _____
	Shorten school day. Specify what hours or courses student will attend: _____

	If student requires home instruction or 1:1 instruction to supplement shortened school day, indicate _____ number of hours of _____ home instruction or _____ 1:1 instruction.
	
	   Indicate location of instruction _____ home _____ school _____
	   _____ other (indicate:)_____

	Provide _____ small-group and/or _____ individual academic support. Indicate frequency: _____ and location: _____
	Provide added adult support during interactions with peers.
	Allow the student to eat lunch in the classroom with a few friends.
	Allow the student to observe other students giving their oral presentations or engaging in an activity before asking the student to give their presentation, etc.
	Reduce exposure to the following settings or activities: _____
	Eliminate exposure to the following settings or activities: _____
Use the Space Below to Indicate Other Non-OCD Anxiety Disorders Accommodations	

Notes:

1. If the student is arriving late to school or avoiding school due to anxiety, the student may require a behavior plan and/or treatment plan.
2. The student may require instruction or training in relaxation techniques and or cognitive interventions.

Attention Deficit Hyperactivity Disorder Accommodations Checklist

General Accommodations

	Use preferential seating _____ close to and/or _____ facing source of instruction.
	Seat student directly facing board or screen if they must copy from it.
	Assist student discreetly with refocusing.
	Alternate quiet activities with opportunities for movement.
	Pause between steps when providing oral directions (for students with slow processing speed).
	Check for comprehension of directions.
	Conference with student after a few minutes or first problem to ensure that they are following directions.
	Break class assignments into smaller units.
	Seat student next to good role model in terms of work pace and sustained focus.
	Tackle difficult concepts early in the day.
	Use more multi-sensory activities.
	Incorporate more large muscle movements or actions in learning activities.
	Establish a safe place or refuge that the student will go to if they need to 'chill' or just get out of the classroom. Indicate location: _____ (to be determined in collaboration with student)
	Allow the child to use calming manipulatives (non-noisy, non-rolling).
	Allow student to use headphones with white noise or familiar music to help filter out distractions.
	Allow student to wear hat to filter out visual distractions when needed.
	Provide a quiet "office" or study carrel in the classroom that the student can go to when he or she is having trouble filtering out distractions.
	Remove distractions like rubber bands or other items that distract the student. Indicate: _____
	Extend time on class work. Indicate: 1.5x: _____ 2x: _____ other: _____

	Ignore minor infractions of classroom rules. Indicate: _____
	Do not penalize student for blurting out.

	Provide staff development program for school personnel:
	     _____ teachers _____ administrators _____ aides _____ related services providers
	     Also include: _____ cafeteria personnel _____ bus personnel
	     _____ other: _____

	Add adult supervision for safety concerns in the following settings:
	     _____ school bus _____ playground/recess
	     _____ field trips

	Provide peer education program for:
	     _____ classmates _____ all students in grade
	     _____ entire building _____ other: _____
	     To be provided by: _____ (name)
	     To be provided by: _____ (date)

Use the Space Below to Indicate Other Attention Deficit Hyperactivity Disorder Accommodations	

Note:

Students with ADHD usually have a number of problems as well as other disorders or conditions. Consult the Executive Dysfunction, Handwriting, Homework, and Testing accommodation checklists as well as checklists for other disorders that the student may have.

Mood Disorders Accommodations Checklist

General Accommodations

	Assist student discreetly with refocusing.
	Provide hard copies of _____ notes and _____ board work.
	Teacher or aide to ensure that all assignments are recorded.
	Teacher or aide to ensure that all materials for assignments are packed.
	Provide an extra set of books to be left at home.
	Reduce or modify homework (see Note 1). Specify: _____
	Eliminate all homework (see Note 1).
	Break large projects down into smaller assignments.
	Conference with the student on a _____ basis to help them stay on schedule.
	Conference with student to find out whether to call on them if their hand is not raised.
	Provide resource room assistance as the last period of the day to enable the student to record and catch up on anything they missed during the first periods of the day.
	Provide resource room assistance as the first period of the day to enable the student to have a more gentle start to their day.
	Do not penalize student for arriving a few minutes late to class (for depressed students with psychomotor retardation, slowing).
	Do not penalize for arriving late to school.
	Have the attendance officer communicate with parents _____ daily _____ weekly.
	Provide added adult supervision for safety reasons. Indicate settings and/or situations: _____
	Have teacher(s) _____ call or _____ email parents on a weekly basis about missing _____ class assignments and/or _____ homework.
	Provide verbal subtitles for students with difficulty accurately reading facial expressions.

	Designate a "safe place" in the building where the student can go to "chill" or take a break. Identify where the student will be permitted to go: _____ (to be determined in collaboration with student)
	Provide staff development program for school personnel: _____ teachers _____ administrators _____ aides _____ related services providers Also include: _____ cafeteria personnel _____ bus personnel _____ other: _____
	Provide peer education program for: _____ classmates _____ all students in grade _____ entire building _____ other: _____ To be provided by: _____ (name) To be provided by: _____ (date)
Use the Space Below to Indicate Other Mood Disorders Accommodations	

Notes:

1. See Homework Accommodations Checklist.
2. Necessary and appropriate accommodations are partly a function of what type of mood episode the student is experiencing. For example, students who are depressed may move slowly and need some accommodations for arriving late to their next class, etc., while students who are hypomanic or manicky have no psychomotor retardation but may have other problems requiring accommodations. Even when students are not symptomatic, however, some problems may persist and schools should be prepared to make accommodations for memory, word retrieval, and executive function deficits.

Asperger's Disorder Accommodations Checklist

	General Accommodations
	Establish consistent routines.
	Use visual organizers for daily routine.
	Place copy of daily schedule on student's desk.
	Point out and highlight any changes in routine on the board and the daily schedule.
	Stand close to student during changes in routine and transitions.
	Provide clear expectations and rules for behavior.
	Teach and reteach behavior rules in all settings.
	Use verbal subtitles for facial expressions or gestures (e.g., say "I am getting frustrated…").
	Assist with cause-and-effect inferences.
	Allow student to leave class a few minutes early to avoid crowded hallways.
	Allow student to wear ear plugs or use other noise-cancelling filters in: _____ hallways _____ cafeteria _____ other: _____
	Designate a "safe place" that the student can go to if they need some "down time" or to "chill."
	Allow "down time:" _____ when student is getting dysregulated _____ after every _____ minutes of work _____ other: _____ Indicate: what the student may do _____ where the student may go _____
	Do not require eye contact.
	Add adult supervision for _____ playground _____ cafeteria _____ school bus _____ other: _____
	Provide written or visual directions when oral directions are provided.

	Provide staff development program for school personnel: _____ teachers _____ administrators _____ aides _____ related services providers Also include: _____ cafeteria personnel _____ bus personnel _____ other: _____
	Provide peer education program for: _____ classmates _____ all students in grade _____ entire building _____ other: _____ To be provided by: _____ (name) To be provided by: _____ (date)

Use the Space Below to Indicate Other Asperger's Disorder Accommodations

Note:

Students with Asperger's have significant impact socially, and often require speech and language services to help remediate social skills deficits. They also face academic challenges. Many of the challenges relate to Executive Dysfunction and cognitive rigidity that impact written expression and comprehension of material. Many students with Asperger's may also have undiagnosed Tourette's Syndrome, Obsessive-Compulsive Disorder, and/or sensory defensiveness that can lead to "melt-downs." Use this checklist in combination with other checklists in this guide.

Medication Side Effects Accommodations Checklist

	Increased Thirst
	Allow water bottles in class or whatever fluids the physician requests.

	Visual Blurring
	Reduce the amount to be read.
	Provide a reader.
	Use books on tape.

	Frequent Urination, Nausea, Vomiting, or Diarrhea
	Provide a permanent pass that the student can use to just leave the room without having to ask.
	Allow the student to sit near the door so that they can leave quickly and without calling attention to themselves.
	Provide hard copies of notes missed while out of room.
	Extend time on classwork.
	Test in a separate location.
	Use flexible scheduling of tests.

	"Rebound" Hyperactivity, Weepiness, or Irritability [2]
	Provide less demanding academic activities during that time.
	Allow more opportunities for the student to move around or engage in activities that are gentle and calming for them during that time.
	Inform parents and prescribing physician to alert them of your observations in case they wish to adjust the in-school timing of the medication.
	Reduce or adjust homework demands if "rebound" occurs after school.

	Loss of Appetite or Reduced Appetite
	Change the student's lunch period, if possible.

[1] Accommodations in this section are organized by type of side effect and not necessarily by type of medication or medication name. These accommodations are not intended to substitute for the advice of the prescribing physician. Schools are encouraged to ask the physician for suggested or necessary accommodations.

[2] As used here, "rebound" refers to hyperactivity, weepiness or irritability that may emerge as a stimulant medication wears off. Not all students on stimulant medications experience "rebound."

	Allow the student to snack in class. Permissible snacks (to be determined in consultation with physician, parents, and student): _____

Increased Appetite

	_____ Permit or _____ ban snacking in class. Permissible snacks (to be determined in consultation with physician, parents, and student): _____

Cognitive Dulling

	Provide word banks for class work, homework, and tests.
	Extend time for classwork, homework, and tests.
	Do not call on student to answer questions unless they raise their hand.
	Provide discreet assistance.

Memory Impairment [3]

	Extend time.
	Provide _____ partial or _____ full notes.
	Do not call on the student to answer questions unless they raise their hand.
	Provide test accommodations such as extended time, short-answer questions with word banks, or alternative methods of assessing the student's knowledge and skills (see Testing Accommodations Checklist).
	Modify test schedule, if necessary, so that student is not studying for more than one test on any given night.
	Prompt student to turn in homework or notes if they forget.
	Have teacher or aide ensure that all important assignments are recorded in agenda.
	Contact parent weekly about any missing assignments.
	If the student forgets to contact teacher(s) about scheduling any make-up tests or if student forgets appointments, teacher(s) will contact the student.

Tics

	Use the same accommodations that you would use for the tics of Tourette's Syndrome if tics emerge as a side effect of a medication.

Sudden "Wildness," Agitation

---

[3] Memory impairment may be part of a disorder, but it may also be a side effect of some medications.

	Notify parents promptly.
	Allow more opportunities for movement.
	Provide more opportunity to engage in self-calming activities.
	Provide copies of notes and board work.
	Provide added adult supervision. Indicate settings: _____
Akathisia [4]	
	Notify parent and allow student to move around or stand.
Use the Space Below to Indicate Other Medication Side Effects Accommodations	

Notes:

1. Many students may require homework as well as classwork accommodations when medication is being adjusted or when medication is failing. Consult the Homework and Testing accommodation checklists.
2. Some medication side effects are potentially dangerous. School personnel need to notify parents promptly if a student's behavior suddenly changes significantly in the directions of depression, wildness, or agitation. If parents consent to direct contact, I recommend schools make contact with the prescribing physician at least once to inquire as to any recommendations the physician may have for their patient. That conversation is an excellent opportunity to ask the physician under what conditions the physician would want to be notified immediately.

[4] Akathisia may be a side effect of some neuroleptic medications. It is experienced as a sense of "inner restlessness" that may appear as anxiety or in more severe cases, as a total inability to sit still.

Sleep Problems Accommodations Checklist

General Accommodations [1]

	Allow the student to _____ start the school day later and/or _____ end the school day earlier. Indicate: _____
	Schedule "heavy" academic courses for _____ mid-morning _____ late morning or _____ early afternoon.
	Ask the student if scheduling a highly motivating class for first period might help them wake up; be guided by their assessment of their situation.
	Allow the student sleep in school. Allow them to sleep for no longer than _____ (amount of time) in _____ nurse's office or _____ other location: _____
	Do not let student sleep in school.
	Provide the student with hard copies of all notes and presentations.
	Have the teacher or aide ensure that all assignments are recorded.
	Extend time on classwork. Indicate: 1.5x: _____ 2x: _____ other: _____
	Extend time on homework. Indicate: 1.5x: _____ 2x: _____ other: _____
	Reduce homework. Indicate: _____
	Extend time on tests. Indicate: 1.5x: _____ 2x: _____ other: _____
	Provide discreet assistance in focusing.
	Allow the student to stand up and move around or walk during class.
	Allow the student to engage in an engrossing activity to offset fatigue.
	Allow the student to _____ go for a brisk walk or _____ run around the gym to offset fatigue.
	Seat the student in a brightly lit area for all academic courses.

[1] Sleep disorders are associated with many disorders. They are also associated with many medications. Consultation with the physician to obtain the physician's recommendations as to which accommodations to provide is strongly recommended.

	Use more self-paced activities.
	Use more multi-sensory learning activities.
	Use more peer activities (e.g., "Think, Pair, Share").
	Provide resource room assistance as the student's first period of the day.
	Provide resource room assistance as the student's last period of the day.
Use the Space Below to Indicate Other Sleep Problems Accommodations	

Checklist for School Personnel and Administrators
Creating a Student-Friendly Environment

	Classroom Environment and Layout
	Post the daily schedule in a spot clearly visible to all students. Include all parts of the daily routine and not just topics or assignments, e.g., include time to record homework assignments and pack up materials.
	Color highlight visual reminders about any changes in routine.
	Use pictorial representations of the schedule for students who can not read.
	Check off each item on the daily schedule as it is completed.
	Have some count-down clocks available for students who have difficulty pacing themselves.
	Post visual cues for upcoming intermediate deadlines where all students can see them. Explicitly call attention to those cues.
	Seat students who need frequent refocusing closer to the teacher and next to a student who is a good role model. If being seated near the teacher will be too distracting for the student because of other students coming up to the desk, seat the student where it is easy to glance over to see if they need help or discreet refocusing.
	Seat students who have visualmotor integration problems so that they can look directly at the board or the presentation area.
	Create different spots in the room where students can go to work if they need to avoid too much visual or auditory stimulation or because they do not want others observing them if they are having a lot of tics. Having a study carrel or "office" that students can go to concentrate on their work will benefit some students.
	Create areas in the room that are shielded and cozy, e.g., a piece of carpeting with bookcases around it for students who may need some "down time" or to remove themselves for a minute or two.
	Make provision for students who tic or for students who cannot handle the close proximity if you cluster desks.
	Allow sufficient pathways and clear areas in the room so that students can get from their desk to the teacher's desk without coming into close contact with other students.
	Establish "checking stations" where students can independently check their work and then go back to their desk to correct it.
	Create a computer or word-processing center.
	Create a music or multimedia center.

© Adapted and modified from Packer, L.E., Checklist for Teachers: Creating a Student-Friendly Environment, 2000.

	Transitions
	Have meetings to point out changes in the weekly routine and enter them on a wipe-off board.
	Use direct instruction during the first week of school using Say, Show, Check to teach students how to make various types of transitions quickly and quietly (e.g., subject-to-subject, sitting-to-lining up, desks in rows to desks clustered).
	Establish and directly teach a routine or system for cueing transitions that involves both visual and auditory cues.
	Establish a routine or system if there is an unexpected change in routine (e.g., fire drill).
	Use repetitions and rituals to foster smoother quicker transitions. If needed, speed up transitions by using techniques such as "beat the clock" and provide rewards for quick and quiet transitions.
	Provide added adult support and a whispered cue to assist students who may have difficulty making a transition due to rituals, cognitive rigidity, or dysregulation.
	Having a larger table or a second desk to go to facilitates transitions for some students. The second desk gives them a change in environment, and may help them leave the previous task behind so that they can start the new assignment.
	Staying Organized
	Use direct instruction to teach "hidden" skills such as how to chunk larger assignments into smaller, intermediate tasks and deadlines.
	Establish a daily routine for when homework assignments are recorded and for when books and materials are packed.
	Establish a daily routine for turning in homework and notes from parents and verbally cue it.
	Provide students with an agenda or visual organizer that allows sufficient space for large, sloppy handwriting and that enables the student to look ahead.
	Establish a homework buddy system for younger students so that they check each other's recording of assignments; make it part of the daily routine. Rotate buddies weekly.
	Establish a buddy system for younger students so they check and help each other pack up necessary papers and materials; make it part of the daily routine. Rotate buddies weekly.
	Establish a routine so that all students immediately mark each piece of paper as either class work or homework and enter the due date. You can use symbols for younger students, "H" and "C" for older students.
	Use color-coded bins for notebooks, texts, and student work of the same content.
	Provide consistent places where materials are kept.
	Provide individual student mailboxes.

	Teach students to routinely highlight important instructions on handouts.
	Teach students to routinely highlight operations symbols on all math worksheets.
	Establish a weekly routine for cleaning out desks.
	Establish a weekly routine for cleaning out folders and book bags.
	Establish a weekly routine for cleaning out lockers.
	Encourage students to bring in an extra supply of pens, pencils, tissues, or whatever they tend to lose or use up most frequently. Schedule some dates on which they all check their "stash" and write notes to replenish. Follow up to see that they have replenished.
	Provide students with daily to-do lists on their desks and teach them to check off each element of an activity as it is completed.
Prosocial Skills	
	Use lavish praise for desirable behavior.
	Establish private signals to cue behavior, i.e., no "public hangings."
	Teach students how to make a "graceful exit" if they need to get themselves out of the room or a situation (Dornbush & Pruitt, 1995, p. 59).
	Provide students who need permission to leave the room frequently with their own permanent pass so that they do not disrupt the class every time they have to leave for a few minutes to get their tics out, calm themselves, etc. Have an agreed-upon place that they will go.
	Preview upcoming events with students and discuss expectations and plans. Role play how they might handle situations.
	For students with high anxiety, discreetly give them a strategy for handling upcoming situations (e.g., "When we go on the field trip tomorrow, you can help me check off each student's name as they get on the bus.").
	Check to determine if the student knows what is expected and how to respond. If not, use direct instruction.
	Teach classroom/curricular units devoted to embracing diversity.
	Have classroom/curricular units devoted to conflict resolution skills and appropriate verbal communications -- rehearse these skills and role play.
	Model ignoring minor infractions and directly teach students to do the same.
	Teach self-advocacy to all students.
	Model and teach respect for individual boundaries.

	Establish one set of rules for the classroom that can work for all students; have the rules allow for accommodations so that students feel that they are all held to the same standard ("Each of us gets what we need and is expected to do what we are capable of."). Teach the classroom rules during the first week of school, with boosters thereafter.
	Have every student in the class have some assigned task or responsibility as part of the community.
	Have some group or class-based rewards and teach the students how they can encourage and assist each other in reaching those goals. Using "Countdown to Extra Recess" during specific academic teacher-directed instructional activities can foster greater focus and participation. Similarly, a Friday "pizza party" if the group turns in over 90% of assigned homework can reward academic productivity.
	Let the sun shine in – particularly early in the day. Dark rooms make it too easy for students with sleep problems, mood disorders, or attentional problems to drift off or to sleep!
	Teach the students how to show you that they are listening to you, keeping in mind that not all students can make eye contact.

Materials and Presentations

	Use worksheets and student planners that allow sufficient space for large, sloppy handwriting.
	Have a supply of paper with vertical guidelines for lining up columns of numbers or graph boxes to facilitate alignment for students with sloppy handwriting or visual-spatial perception problems.
	Check for comprehension of instructions.
	Preview old material and skills thoroughly before introducing new material.
	Introduce one step or concept at a time and check for understanding when doing multi-step projects.
	Provide study guides, outlines, and copies of any overheads.
	Show students a sample of what a completed project should look like before introducing the instructions.
	Use as many modalities as possible. If the student's attention drifts, will they have other cues to help them find out what they missed? Plan each lesson as if you have at least one blind student and one deaf student in the class.
	Have visual cue strips on the student's desk for sequential tasks.
	Teach cognitive cues for sequential tasks (e.g., "Does McDonald's Sell Burgers" for the steps of long division), as well as providing visual cues.
	Break longer presentations into two or three shorter presentations with opportunities for responding or movement between presentations.
	Allocate sufficient time for instructions, repetition of instructions, and individual student assistance.
	Identify goals and subgoals and relate material to subgoals or larger picture throughout presentation.

	Use meaningful examples when introducing new or difficult concepts.
	Use overhead projector to focus attention.
	Monitor student's work pace and work product. Teach students to monitor their pace using count-down clock.
	Provide immediate feedback on performance, including reinforcement for both effort and productivity. With younger students, reinforce effort; with older students, reinforce product.
	Hold props in your hands to encourage students to look at you during presentations. This is particularly helpful for students with autism spectrum disorders.
	Decrease the delays in your presentation so that students are not waiting for you.
	Teach students acceptable delay-filling techniques if they do have to wait for you or their peers.
	Alternate quiet sitting activities with opportunities for more movement.
	Provide worked examples at top of math homework sheets.
Managing Time	
	Use direct instruction to teach students to estimate time needed.
	Use direct instruction to teach students to allow extra time over and above what they think they will need to complete a task.
	Use direct instruction to teach students to keep track of time (e.g., teach them to use a count-down clock, timer, or set an alarm/reminder on a PDA).
	Use direct instruction to teach students to monitor their pace.
	Use direct instruction to teach students to chunk work into intermediate deadlines and to enter intermediate deadlines in their planner.
	Monitor student progress towards intermediate and final deadlines on a frequent basis.
Group Management	
	Establish individual and group rewards and fines for compliance with classroom rules. Teach the reward and penalty system when you teach the classroom rules.
	Use a token system during selected activities that enables the students to earn points towards a group reward.
	Each time a student turns in a homework assignment, give them a ticket with their initials on it that is thrown into a drum or box. On Friday, have a lottery draw so that two students whose tickets are pulled from the box get a free homework pass or some other reward. Start a new lottery draw each week.

	Vary the reward menu for individual students periodically so that students do not satiate on the rewards. Rewards can be activities as well as tangibles (e.g., extra computer time, getting to pick first, etc.).
	Establish a quiet technique for requesting assistance, such as having paper cups on the desks – the student turns the paper cup over to indicate that they need assistance.

Miscellaneous

	Send home the Organizational Skills Survey at beginning of school year for parents to complete and return.
	Send home the Sleep Survey at beginning of school year for parents to complete and return.
	Send home the Homework Observations and Concerns Survey at beginning of school year for parents to complete and return.
	Establish a backup system for students to obtain homework assignments using web, fax, email, etc.
	Provide parents with sufficient instructions and support so that they can assist their child with homework. Do not assume that the parent has the understanding or skills or that the child can clearly explain the assignment to the parent.
	Provide weekly progress reports to alert parents as to any missing assignments or upcoming tests or deadlines.

Building-Wide Ideas

	Have all teachers on a grade level coordinate their classroom rules.
	Implement a building-wide color-coding system for subjects.
	Be proactive on a building level in terms of preventing and dealing with bullying.
	Teach all students relaxation techniques (e.g., breathing relaxation).
	Conduct building-wide programs for students to promote understanding and support of students with disabilities and to embrace cultural diversity.
	Develop a "trick book" for every student in the building, i.e., a book where teachers record strategies or accommodations that were helpful to the student. Each year's teachers can consult the trick book and add to it (Dornbush & Pruitt, 1995, p. 38).
	Have teachers who are designated as Peer Models for how to develop appropriate programs for certain disabilities or behaviors. Let them consult with teachers who are struggling with a student.
	Arrange for staff development programs for different disorders. Include aides, cafeteria personnel, bus drivers, and all who come into contact with children.

	Use the Space Below to Indicate Other Accommodations

Part 3

Organizing Planner for Parents

For Parents: Organizing Your School Concerns

If your child has only one school-related problem or need, you may have no need for a chart, but if your child has a number of issues or problems, you may find it helpful to organize your concerns by using a worksheet planner like the one provided in the next pages. A worked example is provided to illustrate the directions below. You may reproduce the planner as needed to identify all of your concerns.

Start by listing your concerns in Column 1 of the chart.

For each concern, what data can you provide to support your concern? Often, the school's own reports or notes from the teachers will be the support or basis for your concern and request. List those sources in Column 2.

If you think you know the explanation for the problem, list it in Column 3. If you are not sure, leave it blank.

Now that you have identified your questions or concerns, it is time to think about what might help address them.

What accommodations do you think would help? You may already have some ideas as to what your child needs. You can also look over the accommodations checklists provided earlier in this guide to give you ideas. List your ideas in Column 4. If you do not know what would help, leave that column blank.

After you have filled in the planner, go back and prioritize the concerns you listed in Column 1 of the planner. To help you prioritize concerns, ask yourself this, "Which problem do I think is contributing most to academic impairment? Are there any behavior problems that are resulting from my child's disabilities that jeopardize his placement that need to be addressed immediately?"

Once you have prioritized the problems, now prioritize your accommodation requests for those priority concerns. Which accommodation ideas that you listed in Column 4 are easiest to implement and will provide the biggest help? Those will be the ones to raise for discussion if the school does not suggest them or have ideas as to what to do to help. Remember that school personnel have their own expertise. Ask them what they think would work for your child's situation because they know best as to whether an accommodation is readily doable for them or not. The more difficult and time-consuming an accommodation is, the harder it is for the teacher to implement consistently, even though they are motivated to try to help.

If you think your child needs additional assessments to help clarify the nature and extent of any impairment, make a note to request the assessment. As an example, you may wish to request handwriting accommodations, but you may also wish to request that the school's occupational therapist evaluate your child for fine motor, graphomotor, and visualmotor integration skills, as many students with Tourette's, ADHD, and/or OCD have deficits in these areas that may require remediation. Similarly, if your child may need keyboarding, an assistive technology evaluation might be necessary to determine what type of hardware, software, and keyboarding system your child should be provided with or taught.

Planner

Column 1	Column 2	Column 3	Column 4
Concern	Evidence or indications of problem.	If you know what it might be related to, indicate it here:	Possible Accommodations
Reads very slowly	Teacher's notes and report cards all mention problem	• Eye tics are slowing him down. • May be having intrusive thoughts or silent reading rituals that are interfering with reading	• Extended time on reading • Books on tape or someone to read to him • Reduce amount of reading • Does he need assessment on reading comprehension?
His handwriting is horrible	Samples of his work and teacher comments	• Problems with fine motor control and visualmotor integration • Tic interference • Writing rituals	• Reduce handwritten work. Let him use computer • Extended time for writing • Modify worksheets so he has bigger workspace • Don't grade on neatness • Does he need occupational therapy evaluation?
Has melt-downs during homework time	Tell teachers how long homework time is taking and describe his behavior	He's tired and emotional when he comes home from school and says he can't concentrate any more	• Reduce amount of homework • Reduce amount to be written

Planner

Column 1	Column 2	Column 3	Column 4
Concern	Evidence or indications of problem.	If you know what it might be related to, indicate it here:	Possible Accommodations

Resources

Teaching the Tiger: A Handbook for Individuals Involved in the Education of Students with Attention Deficit Disorders, Tourette Syndrome or Obsessive-Compulsive Disorder by Marilyn Dornbush, Ph.D. and Sheryl K. Pruitt. This book is a 1995 classic on accommodations and interventions, and has been translated into many languages.

Tigers, Too by Marilyn Dornbush, Ph.D. and Sheryl K. Pruitt, M.Ed. This book is the long-awaited sequel to Teaching the Tiger and is chock-full of useful tips and strategies for dealing with students with Tourette's Syndrome, Obsessive-Compulsive Disorder, Attention Deficit Hyperactivity Disorder, Executive Dysfunction, and Working Memory problems. This book can be ordered from Parkaire Press, Inc. www.parkairepress.com

Challenging Kids, Challenged Teachers (working title). This book by Leslie E. Packer, Ph.D. and Sheryl K. Pruitt, M.Ed. covers Tourette's, OCD, ADHD, Executive Dysfunction, non-OCD anxiety disorders, and mood disorders, providing case examples and useful strategies for school personnel. The book is currently in press with Woodbine House, and is due out in 2009. Check the www.challengingkids.com web site for updates on its release date.

The Tourette Syndrome Foundation of Canada also has a kit for educators that can be ordered from their web site at www.tourette.ca.

Free Appropriate Public Education for Students With Disabilities: Requirements Under Section 504 of The Rehabilitation Act of 1973. U. S. Department of Education, 2007. This free publication can be downloaded from www.ed.gov/about/offices/list/ocr/docs/FAPE504.pdf or www.tourettesyndrome.net/Files/FAPE504.pdf

For more information by the author of this guide, see the following web sites:
 www.tourettesyndrome.net (Education section)
 www.schoolbehavior.com
 www.challengingkids.com

References

Denckla, M. B. 2007. Executive Function: Binding together the definitions of Attention-Deficit/Hyperactivity Disorder and Learning Disabilities. In *Executive Function in Education*, edited by L. Meltzer. New York: Guilford Press.

Dornbush, M., Pruitt, S.K. (1995). *Teaching the Tiger: A Handbook for Individuals Involved in the Education of Students with Attention Deficit Disorders, Tourette Syndrome or Obsessive-Compulsive Disorder*. Duarte: Hope Press.

Packer, L. E. 1995. Educating children with Tourette Syndrome: Understanding and educating children with a neurobiological disorder. I: Psychoeducational implications of Tourette Syndrome and its associated disorders. : New York State Education Dept., Albany, NY.

Packer, L. E. 1999. A cognitive cue for editing work: the "CLIPS" mnemonic. Unpublished PowerPoint material.

Pruitt, S.K. 1995. "Clueless." PowerPoint presentation and handout on Executive Dysfunction for a staff development course offered by the State of Georgia.